This Essential Oils
Journal Belongs To:

_______________________________

# Essential Oil Inventory

| NAME | USED FOR | DATE OPENED | FAVORITE? |
| --- | --- | --- | --- |

# Essential Oil Wish List

| NAME | USED FOR | PRICE | KID SAFE? |
| --- | --- | --- | --- |

# My Favorite Oils

| ENERGY | CALMING |
|---|---|
| SLEEP | FOCUS/CLARITY |
| WELLNESS | ROMANCE |
| ANXIETY | JOYFUL |

# Testing Out Blends

NAME:



**INGREDIENTS:**

DIFFUSER

INHALER

TOPICAL

OTHER

MY RATING:

NOTES:

# My Oil Ratings

**PURPOSE OF OIL**

NAME:

MY RATING:

**PURPOSE OF OIL**

NAME:

MY RATING:

**PURPOSE OF OIL**

NAME:

MY RATING:

**PURPOSE OF OIL**

NAME:

MY RATING:

**PURPOSE OF OIL**

NAME:

MY RATING:

**NOTES:**

# My Favorite Blends

NAME:

USED FOR:

**INGREDIENTS:**

NOTES:

NAME:

USED FOR:

**INGREDIENTS:**

NOTES:

# My Favorite Blends

NAME:                                    USED FOR:

**INGREDIENTS:**

NOTES:

NAME:                                    USED FOR:

**INGREDIENTS:**

NOTES:

# Lavender Blends

## DIFFUSER BLENDS

**NAME:** SEA BREEZE

2 DROPS LAVENDER

3 DROPS LIME

1 DROP SPEARMINT

**NAME:** COOL DOWN

4 DROPS SPEARMINT

2 DROPS LAVENDER

2 DROPS PEPPERMINT

**NAME:** PEACEFULNESS

3 DROPS LAVENDER

3 DROPS VETIVER

2 DROPS YLANG YLANG

**NAME:** CREATIVE SPARK

3 DROPS LAVENDER

3 DROPS SWEET ORANGE

1 DROP PEPPERMINT

**NAME:** OCEAN BREEZE:

4 DROPS LAVENDER

3 DROPS ROSEMARY

2 DROPS LEMONGRASS

**NAME:** LAVENDAR MINT

4 DROPS LAVENDER

3 DROPS PEPPERMINT

1 DROP VETIVER

**NAME:** CLEAN AIR

3 DROPS LAVENDER

3 DROPS TANGERINE

3 DROPS EUCALYPTUS

**NAME:** MINDFULNESS

2 DROPS LAVENDER

3 DROPS BERGAMOT

2 DROPS ROSEMARY

**NOTES:**

# *Wellness Blends*

## DIFFUSER BLENDS

**NAME:** ENERGIZING

4 DROPS PEPPERMINT

4 DROPS CINNAMON

2 DROPS ROSEMARY

**NAME:** EXTREME FOCUS

4 DROPS BALANCE

2 DROPS FRANKINCENSE

2 DROPS VETIVER

**NAME:** INNER CALM

3 DROPS ELEVATION

3 DROPS BERGAMOT

3 DROPS FRANKINCENSE

**NAME:** TRANQUILITY

3 DROPS LAVENDER

2 DROPS LIME

3 DROPS MANDARIN

**NAME:** LOVER OF LIFE

3 DROPS ROSEMARY

3 DROPS PEPPERMINT

3 DROPS FRANKINCENSE

**NAME:** STRESS BE GONE

3 DROPS LAVENDER

2 DROPS CHAMOMILE

2 DROPS YLANG YLANG

**NAME:** RELAXATION

3 DROPS BERGAMOT

3 DROPS PATCHOULI

3 DROPS YLANG YLANG

**NAME:** ACTIVE LIFE

2 DROPS GRAPEFRUIT

3 DROPS PEPPERMINT

3 DROPS ROSEMARY

**NOTES:**

# *Happiness Blends*

## DIFFUSER BLENDS

**NAME:** CHEERFUL

3 DROPS WILD ORANGE

3 DROPS FRANKINCENSE

1 DROP CINNAMON

**NAME:** INNER PEACE

2 DROPS PEPPERMINT

2 DROPS LAVENDER

2 DROPS WILD ORANGE

**NAME:** WITH PURPOSE

3 DROPS LEMON

2 DROPS OREGANO

2 DROPS ON GUARD

**NAME:** BOOSTER

2 DROPS LAVENDER

3 DROPS SWEET ORANGE

3 DROPS PEPPERMINT

**NAME:** SWEETNESS

3 DROPS BERGAMOT

2 DROPS GERANIUM

3 DROPS LAVENDER

**NAME:** ZONED OUT

2 DROPS ROSEMARY

2 DROPS CINNAMON

1 DROP CLOVE

**NAME:** LAUGHTER

3 DROPS LEMON

3 DROPS TANGERINE

2 DROPS MELALEUCA

**NAME:** MINDFULNESS

3 DROPS LAVENDER

3 DROPS BERGAMOT

1 DROP CLOVE

**NOTES:**

# Well Rested Blends

## DIFFUSER BLENDS

**NAME:** WELL RESTED

3 DROPS JUNIPER BERRY

3 DROPS CHAMOMILE

3 DROPS LAVENDER

**NAME:** WELL RESTED 3

2 DROPS FRANKINCENSE

3 DROPS VETIVER

2 DROPS LAVENDER

**NAME:** WELL RESTED 5

3 DROPS LAVENDER

2 DROPS MARJORAM

2 DROPS ORANGE

**NAME:** WELL RESTED 7

5 DROPS PEPPERMINT

4 DROPS EUCALYPTUS

2 DROPS MYRRH

**NAME:** WELL RESTED 2

4 DROPS CEDARWOOD

3 DROPS LAVENDER

1 DROP VETIVER

**NAME:** WELL RESTED 4

3 DROPS BALANCE

2 DROPS LAVENDER

2 DROPS CHAMOMILE

**NAME:** WELL RESTED 6

3 DROPS LEMON

3 DROPS LAVENDER

2 DROPS PEPPERMINT

**NAME:** WELL RESTED 8

3 DROPS LAVENDER

3 DROPS CHAMOMILE

1 DROP CLOVE

**NOTES:**

# *Autumn Blends*

## DIFFUSER BLENDS

**NAME:** PUMPKIN SPICE

5 DROPS CINNAMON

2 DROPS NUTMEG

3 DROPS CLOVE

**NAME:** SNICKERDOODLE

5 DROPS STRESS AWAY

3 DROPS CINNAMON

2 DROPS NUTMEG

**NAME:** FLANNEL SHEETS

5 DROPS BLACK SPRUCE

4 DROPS STRESS AWAY

4 DROPS ORANGE

**NAME:** SWEATER WEATHER

5 DROPS ORANGE

4 DROPS THIEVES

1 DROP GINGER

**NAME:** CIDER

4 DROPS ORANGE

3 DROPS CINNAMON

3 DROPS GINGER

**NAME:** CHANGING LEAVES

5 DROPS CLOVE

5 DROPS CEDARWOOD

5 DROPS ORANGE

**NAME:** GIVING THANKS

5 DROPS CINNAMON

3 DROPS ORANGE

2 DROPS NUTMEG

**NAME:** AUTUMN BREEZE

5 DROPS CHRISTMAS SPIRIT

2 DROPS CLOVE

1 DROP LEMON

**NOTES:**

# Summer Blends

## DIFFUSER BLENDS

**NAME:** SWEET SUNSHINE

3 DROPS LEMONGRASS

2 DROPS ORANGE

1 DROP PEPPERMINT

**NAME:** SUNNY DAYS

3 DROPS TANGERINE

3 DROPS LEMON

1 DROP PEPPERMINT

**NAME:** HAMMOCK TIME

2 DROPS LAVENDER

2 DROPS CEDARWOOD

2 DROPS WILD ORANGE

**NAME:** CITRUS TWIST

2 DROPS TANGERINE

2 DROPS GRAPEFRUIT

2 DROPS LEMON

**NAME:** SUMMER LOVING

2 DROPS JUNIPER BERRY

2 DROPS GRAPEFRUIT

2 DROPS WILD ORANGE

**NAME:** OCEAN BREEZE

3 DROPS BERGAMOT

3DROPS LAVENDER

3 DROPS ROSEMARY

**NAME:** BEACH MEMORIES

2 DROPS SPEARMINT

3 DROPS TANGERINE

2 DROPS BERGAMOT

**NAME:** SUN KISSED

2 DROPS TEA TREE

2 DROPS LEMON

2 DROPS LIME

**NOTES:**

# Winter Blends

## DIFFUSER BLENDS

**NAME:** WINTER CITRUS

2 DROPS PEPPERMINT

2 DROPS LEMONGRASS

2 DROPS TANGERINE

**NAME:** CLASSIC WINTER

2 DROPS CEDARWOOD

2 DROPS LAVENDER

2 DROPS ROSEMARY

**NAME:** SNOWFLAKE

2 DROPS LAVENDER

2 DROPS LEMON

2 DROPS DIGIZE

**NAME:** HOLIDAY BAKING

2 DROPS CASSIA

2 DROPS VETIVER

2 DROPS LAVENDAR

**NAME:** SNOW DAYS

2 DROPS STRESS AWAY

2 DROPS THIEVES

2 DROPS CITRUS

**NAME:** COZY HOME

2 DROPS BERGAMOT

2 DROPS ORANGE

2 DROPS THIEVES

**NAME:** MOTHER NATURE

3 DROPS PEPPERMINT

3 DROPS LAVENDER

3 DROPS LEMON

**NAME:** WINTER MEMORIES

2 DROPS BERGAMOT

2 DROPS WILD ORANGE

2 DROPS EUCALYPTUS

**NOTES:**

# Spring Blends

## DIFFUSER BLENDS

**NAME:** WELCOME SPRING

2 DROPS GERANIUM

2 DROPS LEMON

2 DROPS GRAPEFRUIT

**NAME:** FRESH & CLEAN

4 DROPS GRAPEFRUIT

3 DROPS PEPPERMINT

3 DROPS CLARY SAGE

**NAME:** SPRING PETALS

2 DROPS YLANG YLANG

2 DROPS PEPPERMINT

2 DROPS JADE LEMON

**NAME:** SPRING CLEANING

2 DROPS LAVENDAR

3 DROPS LEMON

3 DROPS ROSEMARY

**NAME:** SPRING GARDEN

2 DROPS BASIL

2 DROPS PEPPERMINT

2 DROPS LIME

**NAME:** FRESH FLOWERS

5 DROPS CLARY SAGE

3 DROPS LAVENDAR

2 DROPS GERANIUM

**NAME:** MOTHER NATURE

3 DROPS PEPPERMINT

3 DROPS LAVENDAR

3 DROPS LEMON

**NAME:** GOOD MORNING

4 DROPS JOY

3 DROPS LEMON

1 DROP TANGERINE

**NOTES:**

# Holiday Blends

## DIFFUSER BLENDS

**NAME:** DECK THE HALLS

4 DROPS PINE

2 DROPS BLUE SPRUCE

2 DROPS CEDARWOOD

**NAME:** CANDY CANE

4 DROPS PEPPERMINT

3 DROPS BERGAMOT

1 DROP WILD ORANGE

**NAME:** SUGAR PLUM FAIRY

3 DROPS CITRUS BLISS

2 DROPS DOUGLAS FIR

2 DROPS MOTIVATE

**NAME:** OH, HOLY NIGHT

5 DROPS THIEVES

2 DROPS FRANKINCENSE

2 DROPS CITRUS FRESH

**NAME:** SNOW ANGELS

4 DROPS STRESS AWAY

3 FRESH CITRUS

1 DROP FRANKINCENSE

**NAME:** SPICED CIDER

3 DROPS WILD ORANGE

2 DROPS CINNAMON BARK

1 DROP CLOVE

**NAME:** MERRY & BRIGHT

3 DROPS LEMON

2 DROPS DOUGLAS FIR

2 DROPS CINNAMON

**NAME:** GINGERBREAD MAN

4 DROPS GINGER

2 DROPS CLOVES

2 DROPS CINNAMON

**NOTES:**

# Clean House Blends

## DIFFUSER BLENDS

**NAME:** SPARKLY CLEAN

3 DROPS LEMON

3 DROPS PEPPERMINT

3 DROPS EUCALYPTUS

**NAME:** NICE & TIDY

3 DROPS EUCALYPTUS

3 DROPS WILD ORANGE

3 DROPS LIME

**NAME:** FRESH SCENT

3 DROPS LEMON

3 DROPS EASY AIR

3 DROPS LIME

**NAME:** TIDY HOME

1 DROP ROSE

1 DROP CARDAMOM

2 DROPS WILD ORANGE

**NAME:** DECLUTTERING

4 DROPS LEMON

3 DROPS LEMONGRASS

2 DROPS PEPPERMINT

**NAME:** SPRING CLEANING

4 DROPS LEMON

3 DROPS LAVENDER

2 DROPS ROSEMARY

**NAME:** GLOSSY CLEAN

4 DROPS FRANKINCENSE

4 DROPS CYPRESS

2 DROPS YLANG YLANG

**NAME:** HOUSEKEEPER

2 DROPS CINNAMON

2 DROPS CARDAMOM

2 DROPS LEMOM

**NOTES:**

## DIFFUSER BLENDS

**NAME:** CONFIDENT

2 DROPS SPEARMINT

2 DROPS TANGERINE

2 DROPS BERGAMOT

**NAME:** CAREFREE

5 DROPS BERGAMOT

2 DROPS PATCHOULI

2 DROPS LIME

**NAME:** HAPPY

2 DROPS WILD ORANGE

2 DROPS GRAPEFRUIT

2 DROPS CLOVE

**NAME:** INSPIRED

1 DROP ROSE

1 DROP PURIFY

2 DROPS JUNIPER BERRY

**NAME:** FOCUSED

3 DROPS DOUGLAS FIR

2 DROPS LEMON

1 DROP PEPPERMINT

**NAME:** ENERGETIC

2 DROPS PEPPERMINT

3 DROPS GRAPEFRUIT

3 DROPS BERGAMOT

**NAME:** MOTIVATED

2 DROPS ELEVATION

2 DROPS CYPRESS

2 DROPS LIME

**NAME:** PEACEFUL

2 DROPS FRANKINCENSE

2 DROPS WHITE FIR

2 DROPS LAVENDER

**NOTES:**

# Day to Day Blends

## DIFFUSER BLENDS

**NAME:** SLEEP TIME

4 DROPS LAVENDER

4 DROPS CEDARWOOD

3 DROPS CHAMOMILE

**NAME:** ANTI-STRESS

4 DROPS BERGAMOT

4 DROPS FRANKINCENSE

1 DROP PEPPERMINT

**NAME:** ALLERGY BE GONE

3 DROPS LAVENDER

3 DROPS LEMON

3 DROPS PEPPERMINT

**NAME:** CONCENTRATION

4 DROPS LAVENDER

4 DROPS MELALEUCA

4 DROPS FRANKINCENSE

**NAME:** COMBAT NAUSEA

3 DROPS GINGER

5 DROPS PEPPERMINT

1 DROP BALANCE

**NAME:** HEADACHES

2 DROPS FRANKINCENSE

2 DROPS LAVENDER

4 DROPS PEPPERMINT

**NAME:** BREATHE EASY

4 DROPS PEPPERMINT

2 DROPS EUCALYPTUS

2 DROPS LEMON

**NAME:** IMMUNE BOOST

2 DROPS FRANKINCENSE

5 DROPS LEMON

2 DROPS PEPPERMINT

**NOTES:**

# Essential Oil Recipes

NAME:

NAME:

NAME:

NAME:

NAME:

NAME:

NAME:

NAME:

# Essential Oil Recipes

NAME:

NAME:

NAME:

NAME:

NAME:

NAME:

NAME:

NAME:

# Essential Oil Wish List

| NAME | USED FOR | PRICE | KID SAFE? |
| --- | --- | --- | --- |

# My Favorite Oils

ENERGY

CALMING

SLEEP

FOCUS/CLARITY

WELLNESS

ROMANCE

ANXIETY

JOYFUL

# Essential Oil Inventory

| NAME | USED FOR | DATE OPENED | FAVORITE? |
| --- | --- | --- | --- |
| | | | |
| | | | |
| | | | |
| | | | |
| | | | |
| | | | |
| | | | |
| | | | |
| | | | |
| | | | |
| | | | |
| | | | |

| NAME | USED FOR | DATE OPENED | FAVORITE? |
| --- | --- | --- | --- |

# My Favorite Blends

NAME:

USED FOR:

**INGREDIENTS:**

NOTES:

NAME:

USED FOR:

**INGREDIENTS:**

NOTES:

# Essential Oil Inventory

| NAME | USED FOR | DATE OPENED | FAVORITE? |
| --- | --- | --- | --- |
| | | | |

# Essential Oil Wish List

| NAME | USED FOR | PRICE | KID SAFE? |
| --- | --- | --- | --- |
|  |  |  |  |

# My Favorite Oils

## ENERGY

## CALMING

## SLEEP

## FOCUS/CLARITY

## WELLNESS

## ROMANCE

## ANXIETY

## JOYFUL

# Testing Out Blends

NAME:

**PURPOSE:**

INGREDIENTS:

DIFFUSER

INHALER

TOPICAL

OTHER

MY RATING:

NOTES:

# Testing Out Blends

NAME:

**PURPOSE**:

**INGREDIENTS:**

DIFFUSER

INHALER

TOPICAL

OTHER

MY RATING:

NOTES:

# Testing Out Blends

NAME:

**PURPOSE:**

INGREDIENTS:

DIFFUSER

INHALER

TOPICAL

OTHER

MY RATING:

NOTES:

# Testing Out Blends

NAME:

**PURPOSE:**

**INGREDIENTS:**

DIFFUSER

INHALER

TOPICAL

OTHER

MY RATING:

NOTES:

# My Oil Ratings

**PURPOSE OF OIL**

NAME:

MY RATING:

**PURPOSE OF OIL**

NAME:

MY RATING:

**PURPOSE OF OIL**

NAME:

MY RATING:

**PURPOSE OF OIL**

NAME:

MY RATING:

**PURPOSE OF OIL**

NAME:

MY RATING:

**NOTES:**

# My Oil Ratings

**PURPOSE OF OIL**

NAME:

MY RATING:

**PURPOSE OF OIL**

NAME:

MY RATING:

**PURPOSE OF OIL**

NAME:

MY RATING:

**PURPOSE OF OIL**

NAME:

MY RATING:

**PURPOSE OF OIL**

NAME:

MY RATING:

**NOTES:**

# My Oil Ratings

**PURPOSE OF OIL**

NAME:

MY RATING:

**PURPOSE OF OIL**

NAME:

MY RATING:

**PURPOSE OF OIL**

NAME:

MY RATING:

**PURPOSE OF OIL**

NAME:

MY RATING:

**PURPOSE OF OIL**

NAME:

MY RATING:

**NOTES:**

# My Favorite Blends

NAME:                                        USED FOR:

**INGREDIENTS:**

NOTES:

NAME:                                        USED FOR:

**INGREDIENTS:**

NOTES:

# My Favorite Blends

NAME:     USED FOR:

**INGREDIENTS:**

NOTES:

NAME:     USED FOR:

**INGREDIENTS:**

NOTES:

# My Favorite Blends

**NAME:**

USED FOR:

**INGREDIENTS:**

NOTES:

**NAME:**

USED FOR:

**INGREDIENTS:**

NOTES:

# My Favorite Blends

NAME:

USED FOR:

**INGREDIENTS:**

NOTES:

NAME:

USED FOR:

**INGREDIENTS:**

NOTES:

# Essential Oil Inventory

| NAME | USED FOR | DATE OPENED | FAVORITE? |
| --- | --- | --- | --- |

# Essential Oil Wish List

| NAME | USED FOR | PRICE | KID SAFE? |
| --- | --- | --- | --- |

# My Favorite Oils

ENERGY

CALMING

SLEEP

FOCUS/CLARITY

WELLNESS

ROMANCE

ANXIETY

JOYFUL

# Testing Out Blends

**NAME:**

**PURPOSE:**

**INGREDIENTS:**

DIFFUSER

INHALER

TOPICAL

OTHER

MY RATING:

NOTES:

# My Oil Ratings

**PURPOSE OF OIL**

NAME:

MY RATING:

**PURPOSE OF OIL**

NAME:

MY RATING:

**PURPOSE OF OIL**

NAME:

MY RATING:

**PURPOSE OF OIL**

NAME:

MY RATING:

**PURPOSE OF OIL**

NAME:

MY RATING:

**NOTES:**

# My Favorite Blends

NAME:

USED FOR:

**INGREDIENTS:**

NOTES:

NAME:

USED FOR:

**INGREDIENTS:**

NOTES:

# My Favorite Blends

NAME:                                     USED FOR:

**INGREDIENTS:**

NOTES:

NAME:                                     USED FOR:

**INGREDIENTS:**

NOTES:

# Essential Oil Inventory

| NAME | USED FOR | DATE OPENED | FAVORITE? |
| --- | --- | --- | --- |

# Essential Oil Wish List

| NAME | USED FOR | PRICE | KID SAFE? |
| --- | --- | --- | --- |
| | | | |
| | | | |
| | | | |
| | | | |
| | | | |
| | | | |
| | | | |
| | | | |
| | | | |
| | | | |
| | | | |
| | | | |
| | | | |
| | | | |

| NAME | USED FOR | PRICE | KID SAFE? |
| --- | --- | --- | --- |

# My Favorite Oils

## ENERGY

## CALMING

## SLEEP

## FOCUS/CLARITY

## WELLNESS

## ROMANCE

## ANXIETY

## JOYFUL

# Testing Out Blends

NAME:

**PURPOSE**:

**INGREDIENTS:**

DIFFUSER

INHALER

TOPICAL

OTHER

MY RATING:

NOTES:

# My Oil Ratings

**PURPOSE OF OIL**

NAME:

MY RATING:

**PURPOSE OF OIL**

NAME:

MY RATING:

**PURPOSE OF OIL**

NAME:

MY RATING:

**PURPOSE OF OIL**

NAME:

MY RATING:

**PURPOSE OF OIL**

NAME:

MY RATING:

**NOTES:**

# My Favorite Blends

NAME:                                    USED FOR:

**INGREDIENTS:**

NOTES:

NAME:                                    USED FOR:

**INGREDIENTS:**

NOTES:

# My Favorite Blends

NAME:

USED FOR:

**INGREDIENTS:**

NOTES:

NAME:

USED FOR:

**INGREDIENTS:**

NOTES:

# Essential Oil Inventory

| NAME | USED FOR | DATE OPENED | FAVORITE? |
| --- | --- | --- | --- |
| | | | |



| NAME | USED FOR | DATE OPENED | FAVORITE? |
| --- | --- | --- | --- |

# Essential Oil Wish List

| NAME | USED FOR | PRICE | KID SAFE? |
| --- | --- | --- | --- |

# My Favorite Oils

ENERGY

CALMING

SLEEP

FOCUS/CLARITY

WELLNESS

ROMANCE

ANXIETY

JOYFUL

# Testing Out Blends

NAME:

**PURPOSE:**

**INGREDIENTS:**

DIFFUSER

INHALER

TOPICAL

OTHER

MY RATING:

NOTES:

# My Oil Ratings

**PURPOSE OF OIL**

NAME:

MY RATING:

**PURPOSE OF OIL**

NAME:

MY RATING:

**PURPOSE OF OIL**

NAME:

MY RATING:

**PURPOSE OF OIL**

NAME:

MY RATING:

**PURPOSE OF OIL**

NAME:

MY RATING:

**NOTES:**

# My Favorite Blends

NAME:

USED FOR:

**INGREDIENTS:**

NOTES:

NAME:

USED FOR:

**INGREDIENTS:**

NOTES:

# My Favorite Blends

NAME:                                          USED FOR:

**INGREDIENTS:**

NOTES:

NAME:                                          USED FOR:

**INGREDIENTS:**

NOTES:

# Essential Oil Inventory

| NAME | USED FOR | DATE OPENED | FAVORITE? |
|---|---|---|---|
| | | | |



| NAME | USED FOR | DATE OPENED | FAVORITE? |
|---|---|---|---|

# Essential Oil Wish List

| NAME | USED FOR | PRICE | KID SAFE? |
| --- | --- | --- | --- |

# My Favorite Oils

ENERGY

CALMING

SLEEP

FOCUS/CLARITY

WELLNESS

ROMANCE

ANXIETY

JOYFUL

# Testing Out Blends

NAME:

**PURPOSE**:

**INGREDIENTS:**

DIFFUSER

INHALER

TOPICAL

OTHER

MY RATING:

NOTES:

# *My Oil Ratings*

**PURPOSE OF OIL**

NAME:

MY RATING:

**PURPOSE OF OIL**

NAME:

MY RATING:

**PURPOSE OF OIL**

NAME:

MY RATING:

**PURPOSE OF OIL**

NAME:

MY RATING:

**PURPOSE OF OIL**

NAME:

MY RATING:

**NOTES:**

# My Favorite Blends

NAME:

USED FOR:

**INGREDIENTS:**

NOTES:

NAME:

USED FOR:

**INGREDIENTS:**

NOTES:

# My Favorite Blends

NAME:

USED FOR:

**INGREDIENTS:**

NOTES:

NAME:

USED FOR:

**INGREDIENTS:**

NOTES:

# Essential Oil Inventory

| NAME | USED FOR | DATE OPENED | FAVORITE? |
| --- | --- | --- | --- |

# Essential Oil Wish List

| NAME | USED FOR | PRICE | KID SAFE? |
| --- | --- | --- | --- |
| | | | |
| | | | |
| | | | |
| | | | |
| | | | |
| | | | |
| | | | |
| | | | |
| | | | |
| | | | |
| | | | |
| | | | |
| | | | |

| NAME | USED FOR | PRICE | KID SAFE? |
| --- | --- | --- | --- |

# My Favorite Oils

## ENERGY

## CALMING

## SLEEP

## FOCUS/CLARITY

## WELLNESS

## ROMANCE

## ANXIETY

## JOYFUL

# Testing Out Blends

NAME:

**INGREDIENTS:**

**PURPOSE**:

DIFFUSER

INHALER

TOPICAL

OTHER

MY RATING:

NOTES:

# My Oil Ratings

**PURPOSE OF OIL**

NAME:

MY RATING:

**PURPOSE OF OIL**

NAME:

MY RATING:

**PURPOSE OF OIL**

NAME:

MY RATING:

**PURPOSE OF OIL**

NAME:

MY RATING:

**PURPOSE OF OIL**

NAME:

MY RATING:

**NOTES:**

# My Favorite Blends

NAME:

USED FOR:

**INGREDIENTS:**

NOTES:

NAME:

USED FOR:

**INGREDIENTS:**

NOTES:

# My Favorite Blends

NAME:

USED FOR:

**INGREDIENTS:**

NOTES:

NAME:

USED FOR:

**INGREDIENTS:**

NOTES:

# Essential Oil Inventory

| NAME | USED FOR | DATE OPENED | FAVORITE? |
| --- | --- | --- | --- |

# Essential Oil Wish List

| NAME | USED FOR | PRICE | KID SAFE? |
| --- | --- | --- | --- |

# My Favorite Oils

## ENERGY

## CALMING

## SLEEP

## FOCUS/CLARITY

## WELLNESS

## ROMANCE

## ANXIETY

## JOYFUL

# Testing Out Blends

NAME:

**PURPOSE**:

**INGREDIENTS:**

DIFFUSER

INHALER

TOPICAL

OTHER

MY RATING:

NOTES:

# My Oil Ratings

**PURPOSE OF OIL**

NAME:

MY RATING:

**PURPOSE OF OIL**

NAME:

MY RATING:

**PURPOSE OF OIL**

NAME:

MY RATING:

**PURPOSE OF OIL**

NAME:

MY RATING:

**PURPOSE OF OIL**

NAME:

MY RATING:

**NOTES:**

# My Favorite Blends

NAME:

USED FOR:

**INGREDIENTS:**

NOTES:

NAME:

USED FOR:

**INGREDIENTS:**

NOTES:

# My Favorite Blends

NAME:

USED FOR:

**INGREDIENTS:**

NOTES:

NAME:

USED FOR:

**INGREDIENTS:**

NOTES:

# Essential Oil Inventory

| NAME | USED FOR | DATE OPENED | FAVORITE? |
| --- | --- | --- | --- |

# Essential Oil Wish List

| NAME | USED FOR | PRICE | KID SAFE? |
|------|----------|-------|-----------|
|      |          |       |           |

# My Favorite Oils

ENERGY

CALMING

SLEEP

FOCUS/CLARITY

WELLNESS

ROMANCE

ANXIETY

JOYFUL

# Testing Out Blends

NAME:

**PURPOSE**:

**INGREDIENTS:**

DIFFUSER

INHALER

TOPICAL

OTHER

MY RATING:

NOTES:

# My Oil Ratings

**PURPOSE OF OIL**

NAME:

MY RATING:

**PURPOSE OF OIL**

NAME:

MY RATING:

**PURPOSE OF OIL**

NAME:

MY RATING:

**PURPOSE OF OIL**

NAME:

MY RATING:

**PURPOSE OF OIL**

NAME:

MY RATING:

**NOTES:**

# My Favorite Blends

NAME:

USED FOR:

**INGREDIENTS:**

NOTES:

NAME:

USED FOR:

**INGREDIENTS:**

NOTES:

# My Favorite Blends

NAME:

USED FOR:

**INGREDIENTS:**

NOTES:

NAME:

USED FOR:

**INGREDIENTS:**

NOTES:

# Essential Oil Inventory

| NAME | USED FOR | DATE OPENED | FAVORITE? |
| --- | --- | --- | --- |
|  |  |  |  |

# Essential Oil Wish List

| NAME | USED FOR | PRICE | KID SAFE? |
| --- | --- | --- | --- |
|  |  |  |  |
|  |  |  |  |
|  |  |  |  |
|  |  |  |  |
|  |  |  |  |
|  |  |  |  |
|  |  |  |  |
|  |  |  |  |
|  |  |  |  |
|  |  |  |  |
|  |  |  |  |
|  |  |  |  |
|  |  |  |  |

| NAME | USED FOR | PRICE | KID SAFE? |
| --- | --- | --- | --- |

# My Favorite Oils

### ENERGY

### CALMING

### SLEEP

### FOCUS/CLARITY

### WELLNESS

### ROMANCE

### ANXIETY

### JOYFUL

# Testing Out Blends

**NAME:**

**PURPOSE:**

**INGREDIENTS:**

DIFFUSER

INHALER

TOPICAL

OTHER

MY RATING:

NOTES:

# My Oil Ratings

**PURPOSE OF OIL**

NAME:

MY RATING:

**PURPOSE OF OIL**

NAME:

MY RATING:

**PURPOSE OF OIL**

NAME:

MY RATING:

**PURPOSE OF OIL**

NAME:

MY RATING:

**PURPOSE OF OIL**

NAME:

MY RATING:

**NOTES:**

# My Favorite Blends

NAME:                               USED FOR:

**INGREDIENTS:**

NOTES:

NAME:                               USED FOR:

**INGREDIENTS:**

NOTES:

# My Favorite Blends

NAME:

USED FOR:

**INGREDIENTS:**

NOTES:

NAME:

USED FOR:

**INGREDIENTS:**

NOTES:

# Essential Oil Inventory

| NAME | USED FOR | DATE OPENED | FAVORITE? |
| --- | --- | --- | --- |
| | | | |

| NAME | USED FOR | DATE OPENED | FAVORITE? |
| --- | --- | --- | --- |

# Essential Oil Wish List

| NAME | USED FOR | PRICE | KID SAFE? |
| --- | --- | --- | --- |
|  |  |  |  |
|  |  |  |  |
|  |  |  |  |
|  |  |  |  |
|  |  |  |  |
|  |  |  |  |
|  |  |  |  |
|  |  |  |  |
|  |  |  |  |
|  |  |  |  |
|  |  |  |  |
|  |  |  |  |
|  |  |  |  |
|  |  |  |  |
|  |  |  |  |

# My Favorite Oils

## ENERGY

## CALMING

## SLEEP

## FOCUS/CLARITY

## WELLNESS

## ROMANCE

## ANXIETY

## JOYFUL

# Testing Out Blends

NAME:

**PURPOSE**:

**INGREDIENTS:**

DIFFUSER

INHALER

TOPICAL

OTHER

MY RATING:

NOTES:

# My Oil Ratings

**PURPOSE OF OIL**

NAME:

MY RATING:

**PURPOSE OF OIL**

NAME:

MY RATING:

**PURPOSE OF OIL**

NAME:

MY RATING:

**PURPOSE OF OIL**

NAME:

MY RATING:

**PURPOSE OF OIL**

NAME:

MY RATING:

**NOTES:**

# My Favorite Blends

NAME:

USED FOR:

**INGREDIENTS:**

NOTES:

NAME:

USED FOR:

**INGREDIENTS:**

NOTES:

# My Favorite Blends

NAME:                    USED FOR:

INGREDIENTS:

NOTES:

NAME:                    USED FOR:

INGREDIENTS:

NOTES:

# Essential Oil Inventory

| NAME | USED FOR | DATE OPENED | FAVORITE? |
| --- | --- | --- | --- |

# Essential Oil Wish List

| NAME | USED FOR | PRICE | KID SAFE? |
| --- | --- | --- | --- |

# My Favorite Oils

ENERGY

CALMING

SLEEP

FOCUS/CLARITY

WELLNESS

ROMANCE

ANXIETY

JOYFUL

# Testing Out Blends

NAME:

**PURPOSE**:

**INGREDIENTS:**

DIFFUSER

INHALER

TOPICAL

OTHER

MY RATING:

NOTES:

# My Oil Ratings

**PURPOSE OF OIL**

NAME:

MY RATING:

**PURPOSE OF OIL**

NAME:

MY RATING:

**PURPOSE OF OIL**

NAME:

MY RATING:

**PURPOSE OF OIL**

NAME:

MY RATING:

**PURPOSE OF OIL**

NAME:

MY RATING:

**NOTES:**

# My Favorite Blends

NAME:                                    USED FOR:

**INGREDIENTS:**

NOTES:

NAME:                                    USED FOR:

**INGREDIENTS:**

NOTES:

# My Favorite Blends

NAME:

USED FOR:

**INGREDIENTS:**

NOTES:

NAME:

USED FOR:

**INGREDIENTS:**

NOTES:

# Essential Oil Inventory

| NAME | USED FOR | DATE OPENED | FAVORITE? |
| --- | --- | --- | --- |
|  |  |  |  |

# Essential Oil Wish List

| NAME | USED FOR | PRICE | KID SAFE? |
| --- | --- | --- | --- |

# My Favorite Oils

ENERGY

CALMING

SLEEP

FOCUS/CLARITY

WELLNESS

ROMANCE

ANXIETY

JOYFUL

# Testing Out Blends

NAME:

**PURPOSE**:

**INGREDIENTS:**

DIFFUSER

INHALER

TOPICAL

OTHER

MY RATING:

NOTES:

# My Oil Ratings

**PURPOSE OF OIL**

NAME:

MY RATING:

**PURPOSE OF OIL**

NAME:

MY RATING:

**PURPOSE OF OIL**

NAME:

MY RATING:

**PURPOSE OF OIL**

NAME:

MY RATING:

**PURPOSE OF OIL**

NAME:

MY RATING:

**NOTES:**

# My Favorite Blends

NAME:

USED FOR:

**INGREDIENTS:**

NOTES:

NAME:

USED FOR:

**INGREDIENTS:**

NOTES:

# My Favorite Blends

NAME:

USED FOR:

**INGREDIENTS:**

NOTES:

NAME:

USED FOR:

**INGREDIENTS:**

NOTES:

# Essential Oil Inventory

| NAME | USED FOR | DATE OPENED | FAVORITE? |
| --- | --- | --- | --- |

# Essential Oil Wish List

| NAME | USED FOR | PRICE | KID SAFE? |
| --- | --- | --- | --- |